ESSENTIAL OILS
FOR DOGS

40 SAFE & EFFECTIVE THERAPIES AND REMEDIES TO KEEP YOUR DOG HEALTHY FROM PUPPY TO ADULT

MIRANDA ROSS

TABLE OF CONTENTS

INTRODUCTION 5

ESSENTIAL OILS AND BENEFITS FOR DOGS 9

ESSENTIAL OILS..9
BENEFITS OF ESSENTIAL OILS 10

SAFE ESSENTIAL OILS FOR YOUR DOG..............................12

LAVENDER ESSENTIAL OIL 12
BERGAMOT ESSENTIAL OIL 12
ROMAN CHAMOMILE ESSENTIAL OIL 13
HELICHRYSUM ESSENTIAL OIL 13
CARROT SEED ESSENTIAL OIL 13
GERMAN CHAMOMILE ESSENTIAL OIL 13
GERANIUM ESSENTIAL OIL 13
CEDARWOOD ESSENTIAL OIL 14
GINGER ESSENTIAL OIL 14
EUCALYPTUS ESSENTIAL OIL......................................14
CLARY SAGE ESSENTIAL OIL 14

PURCHASE AND STORAGE OF ESSENTIAL OILS 15

APPLICATION TECHNIQUES FOR DOGS.................................18

TOPICAL APPLICATION 18
DIFFUSION 19
ORAL APPLICATION 19

THERAPIES AND REMEDIES FOR DOGS 20

BUG REPELLENT 20
AS EAR DROPS 22
AGAINST FLEAS AND TICKS 24
FOR CLEANING AND SANITIZING................................27
FOR TEETHING PROBLEMS 31
AND ORAL HYGIENE...31
INFECTIONS AND MINOR WOUNDS 33
ITCHY SKIN AND SKIN ALLERGIES 34
MINOR SKIN IRRITATIONS 34
GENERAL WELL BEING 34
THE OLDER DOG 36

SOOTHING EFFECTS OF ESSENTIAL OILS FOR DOGS 38

SPECIAL PRECAUTIONS NEEDED 40

CONCLUSION 42

INTRODUCTION

Pets play a very important role in our lives and are a part of our family. We love them like our own children and want to take good care of them. We want them to live a long and healthy life. A lot of products sold commercially to groom the dog or as health supplements for the pets can have a lot of adverse effects. To prevent any harm to the pet you may want to look at natural and safe alternatives like essential oils.

Essential oils have been around for since ancient times. They are extracted from plants are highly aromatic and concentrated volatile liquid. They have a number of health benefits. If used correctly they do not have any harmful side effects on the animal. They are highly concentrated and have to be used after dilution. This makes a small bottle last for a long time proving to be economical.

Essential oils are absorbed quickly in the body and they act fast. A couple of applications to get rid of fleas is likely to show results. The essential oils work to create a balance in the internal systems of the body. They work on the mind too, thus giving the dog holistic healing.

Essential oils have a soothing and calming effect on the pet, keeping your four legged friends happy and healthy.
In this book you will find a lot of information that you need to start using essential oils and reaping their health benefits.

I hope you enjoy it!

monetary loss due to the information herein, either directly or indirectly.

Respective authors own all copyrights not held by the publisher.

The information herein is offered for informational purposes solely, and is universal as so. The presentation of the information is without contract or any type of guarantee assurance.

The trademarks that are used are without any consent, and the publication of the trademark is without permission or backing by the trademark owner. All trademarks and brands within this book are for clarifying purposes only and are the owned by the owners themselves, not affiliated with this document.

DISCLAIMER: The purpose of this book is to provide information only. The information, though believed to be entirely accurate, is NOT a substitution for medical, psychological or professional advice, diagnosis or treatment. The author recommends that you seek the advice of your physician or other qualified health care provider to present them with questions you may have regarding any medical condition. Advice from your trusted, professional medical advisor should always supersede information presented in this book.

ESSENTIAL OILS AND BENEFITS FOR DOGS

ESSENTIAL OILS

Essential oils are volatile hydrophobic liquids that are extracted from various parts of the plant like the flower, fruit, seed, bark, roots, stem and leaves of a plant. These liquids are highly concentrated and aromatic. It is advisable to use them after dilution.

They are extracted by various methods like steam distillation, solvent extraction, carbon dioxide extraction or manual expression. When we discuss essential oils and their uses we also need to know a little about hydrosols, carrier oils and absolutes.

Hydrosols: These are a by-product when essential oils are extracted by steam distillation.

Carrier oils: These are extracted from the fatty portions, like seed or kernel, of the plant and are used to dilute the essential oil.

Absolutes: These are aromatic substances extracted during the final phases using complex chemical solvents.

The benefits of the essential oils are obtained from their chemical components and can be of great use for humans and animals. Let us see the benefits of the essential oils and how we can use them effectively for our beloved pet, the dog.

BENEFITS OF ESSENTIAL OILS

- They are convenient and easy to use and take very little time to apply. You can also benefit by diffusion of essential oils.
- They are organic. You should purchase only high quality oils to avoid contaminated products. Essential oils when used with the correct dilution are safe for your pet.
- They can be easily diluted.
- They are rich in antioxidants, which remove free radical and improve the immune system.
- They relieve aches and pains in the joints.
- They help solve digestion problems in your pet.
- Minor cuts, wounds, itches and dryness of the skin can be relieved by their use.

- They improve the general well-being of the dog by reducing anxiety and fear and having a calming effect on the dog.

SAFE ESSENTIAL OILS FOR YOUR DOG

Care should be taken while choosing the essential oils to be used for your dog as all oils may not be of benefit. Here is a list of oils that are safe and can be used with proper dilution.

Lavender essential oil

It is the most commonly used safe oil. It helps in soothing and calming the dog. It is used for skin infections, itches, minor cuts and bruises. It has antibacterial qualities.

Bergamot essential oil

Ear infections due to bacterial overgrowth or yeast can be treated with bergamot essential oil. It has antifungal properties and is soothing for the pet. It may cause photosensitization, so avoid taking the pet out after application of this oil.

Roman Chamomile essential oil

This oil is also an absolute essential in your cabinet. It works on the central nervous system of the pet and helps in soothing the nerves. It helps relieve teething pains, muscle cramps and aches in the joints.

Helichrysum essential oil

This too is a very useful oil to keep in the house. It is very therapeutic and acts as an analgesic, relieves inflammation, is regenerative in nature and works to heal scars and bruises.

Carrot seed essential oil

This oil stimulates regeneration and rejuvenation of the tissue and hence is good in healing scars. It works well for dry, flaky skin, sensitive skin that is prone to infections. It is good as a tonic and also helps decrease inflammation.

German Chamomile essential oil

It is good for use on burns, skin irritations and allergies. It is an anti-inflammatory oil.

Geranium essential oil

It is an anti-fungal oil and helps in controlling ear infections caused by fungus. It works in keeping ticks away and for minor skin irritations.

Cedarwood essential oil

It is an antiseptic oil and is useful in many types of dermatitis. It helps in stimulating circulation, repelling fleas, is good for the dog's coat and helps relieve various skin conditions.

Ginger essential oil

Care should be taken to properly dilute this oil, as per instructions, so that it is safe and non-toxic. It helps in controlling motion sickness while travelling and also benefits in conditions like dysplasia, sprains, arthritic pain and digestion problems.

Eucalyptus essential oil

It has anti-inflammatory and anti-viral qualities. It is a good expectorant and helps relieve cold and cough conditions. It is a good flea repellent

Clary Sage essential oil

It sedates the central nervous system and used to calm the nerves of the dog. It has to be diluted properly for use.

PURCHASE AND STORAGE OF ESSENTIAL OILS

A list of things that you should note while purchasing essential oils are given below:

- The oils should be packed in glass bottles that dark and of amber, blue or violet in color.

- The label on the bottle must provide information about the scientific name of the oil, common name, part of the plant used for extraction, the country from where the oil comes, the method of cultivation of the plant.

- The label should mention that the oil is "100% pure essential oil".

- The price is also a criteria. Pure oils are expensive, do not buy the cheap variety as they may be adulterated.

- Sniff the oil before buying. The smell should be strong.

- Avoid buying oil from a company that prices different oils at the same rate, as prices vary depending on the method of extraction.

- Oils sold at supermarkets should be avoided as they are probably expensive, but of inferior quality.

Once you have bought the essential oils you need, proper storage is also important so that the oils retain their quality and therapeutic value. There are various factors that affect the quality of the oil though they do not become rancid.

HEAT AND LIGHT

The color of the oil changes if exposed to direct sunlight for a period of time. This leads to a change in its constituents and therapeutic properties. Essential oils are flammable and though the flash point is quite high, they should be kept away from direct heat.

OXYGEN AND MOISTURE

Oxidation of the oil takes place when and the quality of the oil deteriorates with continuous exposure to air. The oil should not be then used for therapeutic use or topical application

PARTIALLY FULL BOTTLES

The head space in the bottle causes the oxygen present to slowly react with the oil. Once the constituents of the oil separate they do not homogenize again on shaking.

STORAGE

Care should be taken to keep the integrity of the oil intact while storing them. The following points can be kept in mind.

- Essential oils should be stored away from direct heat or light in a cool, dark place
- Plastic bottles should not be used for storage.
- The caps of the bottles should be tightly closed as entry of air or moisture will affect the quality of the oil
- A label with the name of the oil, date of purchase and shelf life written on it should be pasted on each bottle.
- Carrier oils should be refrigerated in summers.

APPLICATION TECHNIQUES FOR DOGS

There are three basic ways to use essential oils for your pet. Correct dilution and application will make sure that you get the maximum benefits and do not cause harm to the pet

TOPICAL APPLICATION

When the oil is applied directly to the affected area, it is said to be applied topically. This method is effective as the oil starts working quickly as it applied on the area of requirement. The amount of oil to be applied can be directly monitored as opposed to inhalation where you cannot be sure of the amount of oil the dog has inhaled.

The oil can be applied by massaging the oil on the affected area after taking a few drops in your hand.
You can also apply the oil by putting the diluted oil in a spray bottle and applying a spritz on the affected area.

The oil can also be added to ointments, balms or shampoos and applied. The pet can be bathed with the shampoo and the affected area will absorb the oils.

DIFFUSION

In this method the oil is diffused into the air with the help of a diffuser and is inhaled by the dog.

The diffuser should be allowed to run for at least forty minutes at a stretch so that there is sufficient time for the oil to diffuse in the air and the dog can inhale an amount that will benefit it. The process should be continued for about a week for the results to start showing.

ORAL APPLICATION

The oil is given to the dog to ingest in this method. The dosage given should be chosen with great care as the oils are very potent due to their high concentration.

THERAPIES AND REMEDIES FOR DOGS

Let us now see the manner in which essential oils are effective in treating and managing used various ailments that plague your dog.

BUG REPELLENT

A number of pests trouble your pet and manifest themselves in their fur or skin. A shampoo that acts as a bug repellant can be used regularly to avoid infestation by bugs such as lice, fleas, ticks and even mange.

Take any mild baby shampoo and mix in it six drops of lavender essential oil for every 30ml of shampoo. Use this while giving your dog a bath. Please, ensure that all the shampoo has been washed off while rinsing. Bugs may still plague your pet and they need special treatment.

LICE

Just like us, dogs can contract lice too. These lice are not contagious to humans. They can give your pet a very itchy skin.

To get rid of lice, two drops of tea tree essential oil and two drops of pine oil can be added to the basic bug repelling shampoo that you have made for your pet. A good lather needs to be worked up while giving your dog a bath. Let the shampoo stay on for a few minutes before rinsing it off. Two drops each of tea tree oil and pine oil should be added to the water used for the final rinse.

The dog's fur has to be combed to take out as many lice as possible. You can apply a blend of olive oil and a couple of drops of pine and tea tree oil and gently massage it on the skin of the pet. This process has to be repeated every alternate day to get rid of the lice.

MANGE

This is generally associated with stray or neglected dogs. There still is a remote chance that your dog might contract Mange especially if its immune system is suppressed. A number of mites are responsible for causing mange which is characterized by itchy skin and patches of skin with hair loss. You will want to treat your pet so that the mites are killed, the lost hair grows back and the immune system recovers.

The animal should be given a bath with the bug repellent shampoo, discussed earlier, to which a few drops of Roman Chamomile are added to increase the soothing effect of the shampoo. This will help in hair growth, soothe the skin and improve the immune system.

A topical application of much diluted Rosemary essential oil mixed with virgin olive oil will help in killing the infection causing mites.

AS EAR DROPS

The ear is a common site of infection in dogs and regular cleaning with a clean cotton swab dipped in a blend of olive oil mixed with a few drops of tea tree and lavender essential oils are recommended. Take care and move slowly to avoid damage to the inner ear of the dog.

If your pet is scratching his ear a lot or there is a discharge which contains pus or blood it is a sign that the pet has contracted an infection of some type or has mites. A blend of olive oil, tea tree oil, Rosemary and lavender oil is effective in this case. A gentle massage behind the ears will help bring the discharge on to the surface and can be cleaned. This treatment should be repeated once daily if badly infected.

To bring out ear wax from the dog's ears put in four drops of a blend of essential oils into the ear canal of the dog and gently massage the ear externally. This will soften the wax in the canal and bring it out when the dog shakes its head. You can then wipe this with a clean cotton ball.

The following oils will be required:
Sweet Almond carrier oil - ½ ounce
Lavender essential oil - 4 drops
Bergamot essential oil - 7 drops
Niaouli essential oil - 3 drops
Roman Chamomile - 2 drops

To relieve pain in the ear Melrose oil is effective. A blend of essential oils that work in ear aches is given below. This should be diluted with vegetable oil before use.

Tea tree essential oil -   1 drop
Lavender essential oil - 1 drop
Roman chamomile oil - 1 drop

Peppermint oil is also useful and has to be applied externally along the line of the ear.

AGAINST FLEAS AND TICKS

All pet owners try really hard to keep their pets safe from fleas and ticks, but your dog magically seems to get them! You certainly need essential oil remedies at hand to try and prevent or treat the fleas and tick problem.

FLEAS

A homemade flea spray can be made by mixing the following and using a spritz over the dog daily to prevent fleas.

Distilled water - ½ cup
Purification essential oil - 6-8 drops
Palo Santo essential oil - 2-4 drops
Thieves hand soap - 1 drop

A few drops of lemongrass oil can be added to the bug repellent shampoo and used to prevent fleas. Lavender oil and a couple of drops of tea tree oil can be blended with olive oil and applied to the base of the dog's tail to prevent fleas. Adding a drop of Peppermint oil while cleaning the floor of the house also acts as a repellent for fleas.

TICKS

Tea tree oil, Melrose essential oil and lemon grass repel ticks. If your dog has caught the ticks their bite can be painful and causes the skin to itch. Here is a remedy to relieve inflammation and any further infection from the tick bite.

Hyssop decumbens oil - 3 drops

Lavender essential oil - 8 drops

Thyme essential oil - 5 drops

Sweet Almond carrier oil - ½ ounce

A blend to prevent ticks can be made by mixing the following:

Myrrh essential oil - 2 drops

Rosewood essential oil - 2 drops

Geranium essential oil -2 drops

Lavender essential oil - 1 drop

Bay leaf essential oil - 1 drop

The above blend is added to 8 ounces of the all-natural shampoo and used to bathe the pet. This will ensure that your dog stays away from ticks. The recipe for the shampoo is shared in the grooming section of this chapter.

Avoiding high grasses while taking the dog for a walk to avoid picking up ticks or walks on the sand to avoid picking up fleas. The dog's bedding can be kept clean by sprinkling a cup of baking soda mixed with three drops of lavender oil and three drops of either oregano oil or tea tree oil. This mixture can be sprinkled on the dog as well.

FOR CLEANING AND SANITIZING

Dogs exude a peculiar odor which permeates the house of the pet owner and can be quite offensive. To tackle this smell a blend of essential oils is generally helpful. It must be kept in mind that this is not a substitute for giving your dog a bath and should be seen only as a stop gap arrangement.

DEODORIZER
A simple recipe for a deodorizer, to keep your mutt smelling fresh, is given here.

Bay leaf essential oil - 3 drops
Black pepper essential oil - 3 drops
Cinnamon leaf essential oil - 5 drops
Caraway essential oil - 5 drops

This can be added to the basic all-natural shampoo and used when needed.

Bergamot essential oil is a natural deodorizer and can be used as a spray to ensure that the house does not have the dog's odor. The blend given below can be mixed and kept in a spray bottle. One spritz of this blend will have your house smelling fresh.

Bergamot essential oil- 8-10 drops

Distilled water- 8 ounces

SHAMPOO FOR THE PUPPY

To keep the pup clean and smelling fresh the following blend can be added to the eight ounce all- natural basic shampoo prepared by you.

Geranium essential oil - 5 drops

Ylang Ylang essential oil - 2 drops

Petitgrain essential oil - 2 drops

Rose essential oil - 2 drops

Roman Chamomile - 2 drops

CLEANSER

A cleanser can be also prepared and stored to be used when needed:

Lavender essential oil - 5 drops

Ravensare essential oil - 5 drops

Grapefruit seed oil - 8 drops

Helichrysum essential oil - 3 drops

Labdanum essential oil -   2 drops

Grain alcohol - 1 teaspoon

Sulfated alcohol - 1 teaspoon

Vegetable glycerin - 1 teaspoon

Distilled water - 1 ounce

Witch Hazel hydrosol - 1 ounce

NOT SO SMELLY DOG

If you just need to freshen up your pet and the smell is not very bad a few drops of essential oils blended with olive oil can be rubbed over the base of the dog's neck, base of the tail and over the tummy area. The choice of oil has to take into consideration the dog's affinity for the smell because, if the pet does not like the smell he will simply go and roll somewhere to gather another smell.

SMELLY DOG

If the dog is smelling quite bad and there is no time to give it a bath you can add oils with a strong smell, like, tea tree oil, eucalyptus oil, rosemary or clove oil. Citrus oils like lime, lemon, grapefruit or orange are also effective.

DRY BLEND

To one cup of baking soda add ten drops of essential oil, which is not disliked by your dog, and let it rest for at least half an hour, so that the powder is infused with the smell of the oil. Sprinkle this powder on your dog and gently massage it in close to the skin. The baking soda will help absorb the oils secreted and neutralize the smell whereas the essential oil will mask whatever smell is left.

Please keep in mind that is solution for bad odor should be used intermittently and not as a substitute for bathing.

FOR TEETHING PROBLEMS
AND ORAL HYGIENE

Brushing your dog's teeth daily is of utmost importance to maintain oral hygiene and healthy teeth. Essential oils can also help in keeping the breath fresh.

FRESH BREATH

The following blend has to be given orally with the help of a dropper, three drops daily. Dog's like this blend and may even drool to prove it!

Coriander seed essential oil - 4 drops
Peppermint essential oil - 6 drops
Cardamom essential oil - 6 drops
Sweet Almond carrier oil - ½ ounce

TEETHING PAIN IN PUPPIES

Drops of the essential oil blend given here can be added to the toy your dog chews to relieve the irritation and pain experienced while teething.

Clove bud infusion oil - 15 drops

Roman Chamomile essential oil - 4 drops

Myrrh essential oil - 6 drops

Sweet Almond carrier oil - ½ ounce

FOR CARE OF THE FUR AND COAT OF THE DOG

A basic all-natural shampoo that has been used in the recipes given above is great for grooming the coat of your pet. This is how it is prepared:

Grapefruit seed extract - 1 ml

Rosemary Antioxidant extract - 1 ml

Cider vinegar - ½ teaspoon

Xanthan gum powder - ½ teaspoon

Distilled water - 4.5 ounce

Decylpolyglucose - 3.2 ounce

Blend these oils in hot water and add xanthan powder later when all the ingredients have blended together. Add the essential oils according to the recipe you are using for various ailments.

After using the bug repellent shampoo to give your pet a bath you can give a gentle application of diluted lavender or rosemary oil all over the coat. Rosemary is good for hair growth and lends a shine to the coat.

Adding geranium essential oil to roman chamomile or lavender essential oil helps in relieving dryness of the skin.

INFECTIONS AND MINOR WOUNDS

The following mix is used by adding it to the all-natural shampoo given above and used:

Helichrysum essential oil - 1 drop

Ravensare essential oil - 4 drops

Labdanum essential oil - 2 drops

Lavender essential oil - 3 drops

ITCHY SKIN AND SKIN ALLERGIES

Mix the following essential oils in 8 ounces of the all-natural shampoo and use:

Rosewood essential oil - 6 drops

Lavender essential oil - 6 drops

Carrot seed essential oil - 2 drops

Geranium essential oil - 2 drops

Roman Chamomile oil - 1 drop

Oatmeal, ground - 1 teaspoon

MINOR SKIN IRRITATIONS

A mix of 2 tablespoons of coconut oil and 10 drops of lavender essential oil when massaged on the dog's coat near the skin, soothes the skin and has a calming effect on the nerves.

GENERAL WELL BEING

To help our dog remain calm and free from anxiety and panic attacks and to promote their general health a few essential blends are shared.

Calming essential oil:

Petitgrain essential oil - 4 drops

Valerian essential oil - 3 drops

Sweet Marjoram essential oil - 3 drops

Sweet orange essential oil - 2 drops

Vetiver essential oil - 2 drop

Sweet Almond carrier oil - ½ ounce

To strengthen the immune system:

2 to 4 drops of the following essential oil are to be massaged on the neck and chest of the pet daily:

Coriander seed essential oil - 2 drops

Thyme essential oil - 2 drops

Bay Laurel essential oil - 2 drops

Ravensare essential oil - 2 drops

Niaouli essential oil - 2 drops

Eucalyptus essential oil - 2 drops

Sweet Almond carrier oil - ½ ounce

To address the stomach ailments peppermint oil can be applied to the paws or rubbed on the belly. Eucalyptus oil is good for relieving coughs and colds and can be inhaled through diffusion.

THE OLDER DOG

As the pet grows older, different issues start plaguing the dog. The eyesight may not be as sharp as earlier, there could be a reduction in the appetite or general alertness. Serious illness like tumors and cancer can also be given some relief with essential oils

INCREASING APPETITE

Dabbing a few drops of essential oils on the paws of your elderly dog and letting it sniff them can boost the appetite. The oils that can be used are; ginger, cardamom, lemon, orange, tangerine, patchouli, spearmint and bergamot.

RELIEVING JOINT PAINS AND ARTHRITIS

A massage of the dog's joints with lemongrass, rosemary or wintergreen essential oil is found to give the dog relief from pain. The massage can be done prior to exercising the dog. A drop of these essential oils can be added to the drinking water of the pet and an improvement can be seen by evening.

IMPROVING EYESIGHT

A blend of essential oils can help the failing eyesight of the elder dog:

Cyprus essential oil - 2 drops

Frankincense essential oil - 2 drops

Rosemary essential oil - 1 drop

Sweet Almond carrier oil - 2 ounces

IMPROVING ALERTNESS LEVELS

Any citrus oil can be applied to the paws of the dog so that it can sniff the oil through the day, to increase alertness levels. Only a few drops should be applied and the oil should be changed to lavender during the night for a calming effect.

HELPING IN CANCER AND TUMORS

Frankincense essential oil is known to be beneficial. Topical application of the oil on external tumors is effective.

SOOTHING EFFECTS OF ESSENTIAL OILS FOR DOGS

Essential oils have various beneficial effects on dogs. They not only treat various ailments but have a positive effect on the general well- being of the animal. Essential oils can be used to calm the frayed nerves, diminish anxiety and panic attacks, promote the immune system and improve the health of the pet.

Let us learn about the essential oils that have a soothing effect on your four legged friend.

LAVENDER

It is an oil that you just can't do without! Lavender oil has anti-bacterial, anti-viral, anti-fungal and anti-inflammatory properties. It helps in maintaining a balance in the internal systems of the body.

It can be used as a mild analgesic and is used to treat minor bruises, cuts and scrapes. Lavender oil soothes the skin if the dog has a sunburn. A tummy rub, every night, with a blend of olive oil keeps the dog happy and calm. It is also beneficial in calming a dog displaying neurotic behavior.

ROSEMARY ESSENTIAL OIL

This essential oil has strong anti-bacterial, anti-viral and anti-fungal properties. It helps in relieving muscle stiffness and joint pains. It is great in elevating the mood of the pet and improves the immune system of the animal.

ROMAN CHAMOMILE ESSENTIAL OIL

This oil has sedative and analgesic properties that soothe and calm the pet. Give your dog a tummy rub at night with a mix of lavender, olive and roman chamomile oil to have a calming effect and help the dog sleep better. If the dog has had a big meal this oil will relieve flatulence.

PEPPERMINT AND FENNEL ESSENTIAL OIL

Both these oils are good for the digestive system of the pet. Peppermint oil is good for expelling parasites and hence a tummy rub with this oil at night is useful in deworming the dog. It is also an analgesic and used to relieve tummy aches. To help relieve stomach cramps, flatulence and bloating due to gas build up these oils come in handy.

SPECIAL PRECAUTIONS NEEDED

To reap the various benefits of essential oils you should be well informed about the essential oils that you use for your pet. They should be used with proper dilution, as instructed.

Essential oils can increase toxicity in the body, give rise to allergies, damage the liver or kidneys and in extreme cases prove to be fatal. To avoid harming your pet, here are a few precautions that you should take before using essential oils for your dog:

- While purchasing the essential oil choose one that is labelled 100% pure to ensure good quality. Adulterated oils can cause more harm than good.
- Choose the one that is listed as a safe essential oil.
- To avoid toxicity ensure proper dilution of the oil.
- Dilution should be increased for an older pet, puppy or one in poor health.
- Dilution has to be altered to suit the size of the dog.

- No essential oil should be administered to a dog suffering from seizures.
- While applying the oils care should be taken to avoid the areas near the eyes, anus or genitals as this can cause irritation.
- The behavior of the pet should be monitored closely while starting the use of a new oil.
- Stop the use of the oil if the dog feels sick and does not behave like its normal self.
- The sun should be avoided if the oil applied is photosensitive.
- A patch test should be conducted to check for allergies.
- Essential oils should be kept away from direct heat, light and ignition source.
- All essential oils should be kept away from the reach of pets.

CONCLUSION

Essential oils are nature's gift. We can make the maximum use of this wonderful gift by using them with precaution and being well informed of the properties of each oil.

This book has endeavored to share with you the basics of essential oils, the benefits they impart, how to purchase and store these oils, how to apply these oils and most importantly, the various ailments that can be treated by these oils.

Regular use of essential oils with your pet will help in keeping your dog in good health both mentally and physically. You will observe that the dog is calmer and happier due to the soothing effects of the oils.

Diffusion of essential oils benefits the whole family. These oils elevate the mood and have a calming effect. They are safe to use due to their organic nature. Care should be taken to purchase pure oils and use them with dilution to avoid any adverse effect.

When used properly, you will find that these essential oils go a long way in treating your dog with home remedies and are simple and easy to use.

Hope you and your pet gain the maximum benefits and stay healthy and happy with the use of these fine essential oils.

Should you find this book extremely of help, sharing it with your friends and loved ones will be greatly valued.
Thank you and good luck!

FROM THE AUTHOR

I would like to ask you for a small favor. Book reviews are very important for other dog enthusiasts like you. If you found this book useful, please take the time to share your thoughts and leave a comment under my book.

Thank You!

Check Out My Other Books

Bellow you will find my other books that are popular on Kindle.

Health & beauty:

Body Scrubs: 30 Organic Homemade Body And Face Scrubs, The Best All-Natural Recipes For Soft, Radiant And Youthful Skin

Natural Hair Care Guide: How To Stop Hair Loss And Accelerate Hair Growth In A Natural Way, Get Strong, Healthy And Shiny Hair Without Chemicals

Essential Oils Guide: The Ultimate Guide To Essential Oils For Weight Loss, Stress Relief, Aromatherapy, Beauty Care, Easy Recipes For Health & Beauty

<u>Anti-Aging Skin Care Secrets: Younger Skin Without Scalpel And Botox. Discover How To Rejuvenate Your Skin Quickly And Maintain A Youthful Appearance</u>

Growing orchids:

<u>Orchids: Growing Orchids Made Easy And Pleasant. The Most Common Errors In The Cultivation Of Orchids. Let Your Orchids Grow For Many Years</u>

<u>Orchids Care For Hobbyists: The Advanced Guide For Orchid Enthusiasts</u>

<u>Phalaenopsis Orchids Care: 30 Most Important Things To Remember When Growing Phalaenopsis Orchids, How To Give The Best Life To Your Plants</u>

<u>Orchids Care Bundle (Orchids + Orchids Care For Hobbyists): Growing Orchids Made Easy And Pleasant + The Advanced Guide For Orchid Enthusiasts</u>

<u>Phalaenopsis Orchids Box Set 2 in 1: Phalaenopsis Orchids Care + Orchids Care For Hobbyists</u>

Orchids Care Bundle 3 in 1: Orchids + Orchids Care For Hobbyists + Phalaenopsis Orchids Care

Speed Reading Guide For Beginners:

Speed Reading Guide For Beginners: Get Your Fast Reading Skill The Easy Way. Simple Techniques To Increase Your Reading Speed In Less 24 Hours

You can simply search for the titles on the Amazon website to find them. Best regards!

Printed in Great Britain
by Amazon